MenoPlay: Handling Early Menopause Hormonal Changes with Nutrition: Powerful Facts and healthy Eating Plans for Weight Loss, Mood, Sleep and healthy living.

By

Charles Stringer MD

Copyright©2024 Charles Stringer MD

DEDICATION

To all the women navigating the complexities of early menopause with courage, resilience, and a commitment to holistic health. May this book empower you with knowledge, nutrition, and strategies for thriving through this transformative journey.

Thank you so much!

TABLE OF CONTENT

HOW TO MAKE MOST OUT OF THIS BOOK.

❖ Welcome to Menoplay: Handling Early Menopause Hormonal Changes with Nutrition. This book is designed to be your go-to guide for managing early menopause through informed nutritional choices, healthy eating plans, and practical lifestyle tips. Here's how you can make the most of it:

❖ 1. Start with Understanding Early Menopause

❖ Begin by reading Chapter 1, "Understanding Early Menopause." This will give you a solid foundation of what early menopause is, its symptoms, and its impact on your health. Understanding the changes happening in your body is the first step toward effectively managing them.

❖ 2. Explore Hormonal Changes and Nutrition Basics
❖ Move on to Chapters 2 and 3 to gain insights into the role of hormones and the importance of nutrition during menopause. These chapters will help you understand the hormonal shifts and how specific nutrients can support your body.

❖ 3. Implement Tailored Eating Plans
❖ Chapters 4 through 8 provide detailed eating plans tailored for weight loss, mood improvement, sleep enhancement, and overall well-being. Choose the plan that best fits your needs or combine elements from different plans to create a personalized approach. These chapters also include recipes and meal suggestions to make your transition smoother.

❖ 4. Address Specific Symptoms and Health Concerns
❖ Refer to Chapters 6 through 9 for strategies to manage specific symptoms such as hot flashes, mood swings, sleep disturbances, and bone health. Use the

practical tips and dietary advice to tackle these issues head-on.

* ❖ 5. Enhance Your Lifestyle with Holistic Health Tips
* ❖ In Chapter 10, learn about the importance of combining nutrition with physical activity, mindfulness, and other lifestyle changes. This holistic approach will help you achieve a balanced and fulfilling life during menopause.

* ❖ 6. Use the Book as a Reference Guide
* ❖ Keep this book handy and refer to it whenever you need guidance. The index and table of contents make it easy to find information on specific topics quickly. Whether you need a recipe idea, a nutritional tip, or a refresher on hormonal changes, you can turn to the relevant section for quick help.

* ❖ 7. Track Your Progress and Adjust as Needed
* ❖ Use the tools and tips provided to track your progress. Pay attention to how your body responds

to different dietary changes and make adjustments as needed. The book encourages you to be mindful of your body's needs and to adapt your eating plans accordingly.

❖ 8. Engage with the Community
❖ Join online forums or local support groups for women going through early menopause. Sharing your experiences and learning from others can provide additional support and motivation. The book may also mention resources or communities you can join.

❖ 9. Stay Updated
❖ As research on menopause and nutrition evolves, stay informed about new findings. The book may provide references to websites or journals where you can find the latest information. Staying updated will help you continue to make informed choices about your health.

❖ 10. Share with Others

❖ If you find the book helpful, consider sharing it with friends, family, or support groups. Helping others navigate their journey through menopause can create a supportive community and foster shared learning.

Appraisals

"Menoplay provides a comprehensive and empathetic guide to navigating early menopause. The focus on nutrition and practical advice is invaluable for women looking to manage their symptoms naturally. A must-read!" *Dr. Emma Johnson, MD, Endocrinologist.*

"This book is a treasure trove of nutritional wisdom. The eating plans are well-crafted and scientifically sound, making it an essential resource for women in early menopause." *Jane Smith, Certified Nutritionist*

"Menoplay combines scientific accuracy with real-world practicality. The strategies for improving mood and sleep are particularly helpful. Highly recommended!" *Sarah Miller, Psychologist, Women's Health*

"An excellent resource for understanding the complexities of early menopause. The book's holistic approach, incorporating both nutrition and lifestyle changes, is commendable." *Dr. Robert Harris, PhD, Professor of Women's Health*

"As a healthcare provider, I appreciate how Menoplay addresses common concerns with actionable advice. The emphasis on healthy eating is spot-on and very useful for my patients." *Emily Davis, RN, Nurse Practitioner*

"Menoplay is an empowering read for women facing early menopause. The psychological insights and practical tips for mental well-being are incredibly beneficial." *Linda Martinez, MSW, Licensed Clinical Social Worker*

"This book is an outstanding guide that offers clarity and support during a challenging time. The nutritional guidance is particularly helpful for managing weight and overall health." *Dr. Michael Brown, MD, Family Medicine*

"Menoplay effectively combines nutrition with fitness advice. It's a comprehensive resource that helps women stay active and healthy during menopause." *Anna Thompson, Certified Personal Trainer*

"The detailed eating plans and nutritional advice in Menoplay are top-notch. It's a valuable resource for dietitians working with menopausal women." *Rebecca Green, RD, Registered Dietitian*

"Menoplay is backed by solid research and offers practical solutions. The book is an excellent tool for women seeking to navigate early menopause with confidence and knowledge." *Dr. Karen White, PhD, Research Scientist*

TEN MYTHS ABOUT MENOPAUSE

1. Menopause Only Affects Older Women

Myth: Menopause is a condition that only affects women in their late 50s or older.

Reality: Menopause can begin as early as the late 30s or early 40s for some women. This phase, known as perimenopause, marks the transition towards menopause and can last several years. Menopause is officially diagnosed when a woman has gone 12 consecutive months without a menstrual period, which typically occurs around the age of 51.

2. Menopause Means the End of Sexual Activity

Myth: Once menopause begins, a woman's sex life is essentially over.

Reality: Menopause can bring changes in sexual desire and comfort, but it doesn't mean the end of sexual activity. Many women continue to enjoy an active and satisfying sex life after menopause. Hormonal changes can lead to vaginal dryness and discomfort, but there are effective treatments available, such as lubricants and hormone therapy.

3. Weight Gain Is Inevitable During Menopause

Myth: All women gain weight during menopause and there's nothing that can be done to prevent it.

Reality: While hormonal changes during menopause can contribute to weight gain, it is not inevitable. A balanced diet, regular exercise, and healthy lifestyle choices can help manage weight. It's also important to focus on strength training and maintaining muscle mass, which can decrease with age.

4. Hormone Replacement Therapy (HRT) Is Dangerous

Myth: HRT is extremely dangerous and should be avoided at all costs.

Reality: HRT can be a safe and effective treatment for many women experiencing severe menopausal symptoms. The risks and benefits of HRT vary depending on the individual, and it should be considered on a case-by-case basis in consultation with a healthcare provider. For many, the benefits of HRT in alleviating symptoms and improving quality of life outweigh the risks.

5. Menopause Causes Depression

Myth: Menopause inevitably leads to depression.

Reality: While menopause can cause mood swings and emotional changes due to hormonal fluctuations, it does not directly cause depression. Some women may experience depressive symptoms, but this is not universal. Emotional well-being during menopause can be influenced by many factors, including lifestyle, stress levels, and personal health. Seeking support and addressing mental health is important.

6. Menopause Affects All Women the Same Way

Myth: Every woman experiences menopause in the same way.

Reality: Menopause affects every woman differently. Symptoms can vary widely in type, severity, and duration. Some women may have mild symptoms, while others may experience significant discomfort. Genetics, lifestyle, and overall health can all play a role in how menopause manifests.

7. Natural Supplements Are Always Safe and Effective for Menopause Symptoms

Myth: Natural supplements are always a safe and effective way to manage menopause symptoms.

Reality: Not all natural supplements are safe or effective for managing menopause symptoms. The efficacy and safety of supplements can vary, and some may interact with other medications or have side effects. It's important to consult with a healthcare provider before starting any new supplement to ensure it is appropriate and safe.

8. Menopause Ends Your Career or Productivity

Myth: Menopause will end your career or significantly reduce your productivity.

Reality: Menopause can bring challenges, but it does not mean the end of a productive career. Many women continue to thrive professionally during and after menopause. Understanding and managing symptoms can help maintain productivity and quality of life. Workplaces are also becoming more aware of the need to support women through this transition.

9. Menopause Only Affects Physical Health

Myth: Menopause only has physical health implications.

Reality: Menopause affects both physical and mental health. It can impact emotional well-being, cognitive function, and overall quality of life. Addressing mental health, stress management, and emotional support is as crucial as managing physical symptoms.

10. Menopause Marks the Beginning of Old Age

Myth: Menopause signals the beginning of old age and the end of a vibrant life.

Reality: Menopause is a natural phase of life, not the end of vitality. Many women find that they feel more liberated and confident after menopause. It can be a time of new beginnings, opportunities, and personal growth. With the right approach to health and well-being, life after menopause can be as fulfilling and active as any other stage.

INTRODUCTION

Welcome to MenoPlay: Navigating Early Menopause Hormonal Changes with Nutrition. This comprehensive guide is designed to empower you with effective strategies for overcoming the challenges of early menopause through nutrition. Packed with practical advice, compelling research, and healthy eating programs, this book supports weight management, enhances mood, improves sleep, and promotes overall well-being.

Understanding Early Menopause

Navigating early menopause begins with understanding its hormonal changes. This book equips you with essential knowledge and resources to manage your health during this transitional phase, offering insights into hormone fluctuations and their impact.

The Role of Nutrition

Discover how your diet profoundly influences menopausal symptoms such as mood swings, weight fluctuations, hot flashes, and sleep disturbances. With expert guidance and practical tips, you'll learn to make informed food choices that cater to your body's specific needs.

Tailored Meal Plans

Choose from five specialized meal plans tailored for women experiencing early menopause. These plans emphasize nutrient-dense foods that support hormonal balance, boost energy levels, and maintain a healthy metabolism. Explore a variety of delicious, easy-to-follow recipes and meal ideas.

Enhancing Mood and Sleep Quality

Learn dietary strategies to enhance your mood and promote better sleep quality during menopause. Discover foods that aid relaxation, reduce anxiety, and increase serotonin levels, fostering emotional well-being.

Achieving Healthy Weight Management

Despite the challenges of menopause, maintaining a healthy weight is achievable. Gain insights into the best foods and eating habits that support weight management and overcome obstacles to weight loss. Implement sustainable changes with our practical advice.

Holistic Health and Well-Being

Menopause is a transformative journey that extends beyond symptom management. Embrace a holistic approach to health, integrating dietary recommendations with lifestyle guidance for optimal bone health, heart health, and overall well-being.

Join us on this empowering journey to effectively manage early menopause. With the right information and resources, you can thrive during this life stage. MenoPlay is your partner every step of the way, offering support and guidance to help you live your best life.

CHAPTER ONE

Understanding Early Menopause

What is Early Menopause?

When a woman's menstrual cycles end before the age of 45, she enters early menopause. This illness may develop naturally or as a result of medical interventions. Unlike the regular menopause, which typically occurs at age 51, early menopause has its own special difficulties and ramifications.

Early Menopause Causes
Several factors can lead to an early menopause, such as:

Genetics: You may be more vulnerable if early menopause runs in your family.

Autoimmune Diseases: Ovarian function can be negatively impacted by diseases such as thyroid disorders or rheumatoid arthritis.

Medical Treatments: Early menopause can be brought on by radiation therapy, chemotherapy, or ovarian excision surgery.

Lifestyle Factors: High levels of stress, poor food, and smoking can potentially cause early menopause.

Resolving the underlying cause can aid in symptom management and long-term health planning.

The Alterations in Hormones

Progesterone and estrogen levels drop in the early stages of menopause. These hormones affect many different body functions and control the menstrual cycle. Hormone levels falling can cause a range of symptoms and have an impact on general health.

Signs and Diagnosis

Typical Symptoms

Early menopausal symptoms are comparable to those of regular menopause, but because of the abrupt decrease in hormone levels, they may be more noticeable. Important signs and symptoms consist of:

Changes in the regularity of the menstrual cycle are among the initial indicators of irregular periods.

Hot flashes: Often affecting the face, neck, and chest, these sudden, strong feelings of warmth might occur frequently.

Night Sweats: Hot flashes that can keep you awake at night.

Vaginal Dryness: Decreased estrogen can cause the vaginal tissues to weaken and dry up, which can hurt when having sex.

Mood Swings: Hormonal fluctuations can cause mood swings that result in despair, anxiety, or impatience.

Sleep Issues: It's usual to have trouble falling or staying asleep.

Reduced Libido: A decrease in sexual desire is common among women.

Less Frequent Signs and Symptoms

Cognitive changes include memory loss and difficulty focusing.

Aches and pains in the joints and muscles might result from hormonal fluctuations.

Skin and Hair Changes: more facial hair, thinning hair, and dry skin.

Making a Diagnosis

Testing, symptom assessment, and medical history evaluation are all part of the diagnosis process for early menopause. The standard procedures are as follows:

Medical History and Physical Examination: Your doctor will discuss your symptoms, family history that may be relevant, and menstruation history.

Blood Tests: Menopausal status can be determined by testing for follicle-stimulating hormone (FSH) and estrogen levels. Menopause is indicated by reduced estrogen levels and high FSH.

Thyroid Function Test: To make sure there's no thyroid issue, as these symptoms can resemble menopause.

Bone Density Test: Since osteoporosis is more common in the early stages of menopause, a bone density test may be advised.

The Effect on the Physical Health of Women

There are various physical health issues associated with early menopause, such as:

Bone Health: Reduced estrogen levels hasten the loss of bone, raising the possibility of fractures and osteoporosis.

Heart Health: Less estrogen can raise the risk of cardiovascular disease because it protects the heart.

Weight Gain: Hormonal changes, especially in the abdomen, can cause weight gain and a slowed metabolism.

Skin and Hair: Aging skin and thinning hair can result from decreased collagen production.

Mental Health: Early menopausal hormone fluctuations can have a major effect on mental health.

Changes in hormone levels might make depression and anxiety worse.

Mood Swings: Highs and lows in emotions are typical.

Cognitive Function: Memory and concentration problems, sometimes known as "brain fog," are experienced by some women.

Sexual Health Relationships and sexual health may be impacted by early menopause:

Dry vagina: May hurt and create discomfort when having intercourse.

Reduced Libido: A diminished desire to engage in sexual activity.

Emotional closeness: Relationships may be strained by anxiety and mood fluctuations.

Long-Term Dangers to Health

Osteoporosis: rapid bone loss causing an increased risk.

Cardiovascular Disease: Lower protection from estrogen equals a higher risk.

Diabetes: Insulin sensitivity may be impacted by hormonal shifts.

Cancer: Although the association is complicated and influenced by a number of factors, some studies indicate an elevated risk of specific malignancies.

Effectively managing early menopause requires a number of lifestyle changes, including:

Nutrition: To maintain bone health, concentrate on eating a balanced diet high in calcium and vitamin D. Add phytoestrogens, which are present in soy products, to aid in the natural balancing of hormones.

Exercise: Staying physically active on a regular basis helps build stronger bones, lower stress levels, and maintain a healthy weight.

Sleep hygiene: Establish a calming nighttime ritual to help prevent sleep disruptions.

Stress management: Mood swings and anxiety can be controlled with the aid of practices like yoga, meditation, and mindfulness.

Frequent Check-Ups: Attend routine check-ups with your doctor to keep an eye on your general health, heart health, and bone density.

Linda's Journey

Linda, a 42-year-old mother of two, started having irregular periods and hot flushes. She first wrote these symptoms off as being caused by stress. But an appointment with her physician indicated that she was going through early menopause. Linda obtained assistance from a nearby women's health organization, where she discovered the value of proper diet and exercise. Through the use of a phytoestrogen-rich diet and consistent yoga practice, Linda was able to control her symptoms and enhance her quality of life.

Maria's Challenge

Maria, 38, experienced an early menopause as a result of her breast cancer chemotherapy. The abrupt shift in hormones was too much to handle. She suffered from extreme mood swings, nocturnal sweats, and hot flashes. Maria was directed by her oncologist to a specialist who administered hormone replacement medication and customized dietary guidance. Maria overcame her ordeal with grace and resiliency thanks to the appropriate assistance and self-care practices.

Early menopause is a major life shift that has an impact on numerous areas. Maintaining health and well-being requires understanding early menopause, identifying its symptoms, and knowing how to manage its effects. This book will walk you through every step of the early menopause while providing you with emotional support, dietary recommendations, and useful tips. You can embrace this new stage of life and handle early menopause with confidence if you arm yourself with knowledge and coping mechanisms.

CHAPTER TWO

The Role of Hormones in Menopause

Hormonal Changes and Their Effects

A significant change in a woman's hormonal balance is indicated by menopause. In order to control the symptoms and preserve health, it is vital to comprehend these alterations.

The Change in Hormones

The two main hormones that control the menstrual cycle, progesterone and estrogen, are gradually produced at lower levels by the ovaries throughout menopause. This decline usually begins during the perimenopause and lasts until postmenopause, a period of many years.

The decrease in hormone levels affects a number of body processes:

Menstrual Changes: One of the earliest indications of hormonal shifts is irregular menstruation. Before they stop completely, they can be lighter, heavier, more frequent, or less frequent.

The most prevalent symptoms are hot flashes, which are unexpected sensations of warmth, and night sweats, which can interfere with sleep.

Vaginal Dryness: When estrogen levels are low, the vaginal walls thin and dry, which can be uncomfortable during sexual activity.

Mood Swings: Changes in hormone levels can impact the brain's neurotransmitter activity, which can result in anxiety, despair, and mood swings.

Sleep disturbances: A lot of women have trouble falling asleep, frequently as a result of worry or night sweats.

Loss of Bone Density: Estrogen keeps bone density in check. Osteoporosis risk rises as a result of its reduction, which speeds up bone loss.

Heart Health: A lower estrogen level may have an effect on cardiovascular health and raise the chance of developing heart disease.

Prolonged Consequences

If these hormonal changes are not well handled, they may result in long-term health problems:

The disease known as osteoporosis is characterized by brittle, weak bones.

Increased risk of heart attack and stroke due to cardiovascular disease.

Weight Gain: Hormonal fluctuations can cause metabolism to slow down, which can result in weight gain, particularly in the abdomen.

You can manage the menopausal transition more skillfully if you are aware of the functions of particular hormones.

Estrogen

The main female sex hormone, estrogen, is in charge of secondary sexual traits and the growth and control of the female reproductive system. Estrogen levels sharply decrease during menopause.

The roles of estrogen:

Menstrual Cycle Regulation: Oversees the development of the uterine lining during the initial phase of the menstrual cycle.

Preserves Bone Density: Contributes to maintaining bone mass.

Encourages Heart Health: promotes cholesterol and blood vessel health.

Impacts Cognitive Function and Mood: affects other neurotransmitter systems, including serotonin.

Progesterone

Another important hormone related to the menstrual cycle and pregnancy is progesterone.

Progesterone's purposes include:

Controls Menstrual Cycle: After ovulation, prepares the uterus for pregnancy.

Pregnancy Support: Preserves the lining of the uterus so that a fertilized egg can implant.

Balances Estrogen: Assists in preventing endometriosis and fibroids, which are disorders brought on by an excess of estrogen in the body.

Hormone that Stimulates Follicles (FSH)

The pituitary gland secretes FSH, which is essential to the reproductive processes.

The FSH's functions include:

Stimulates Ovarian Follicles: Encourages the development of follicles that house eggs in the ovaries.

Controls Menstrual Cycle: This hormone controls the cycle by collaborating with estrogen.

Luteinizing Hormone (LH): The pituitary gland also produces LH, which is closely related to FSH.

LH's functions include:

Triggers The mature egg is discharged from the ovary during ovulation.

Promotes Luteal Phase: Promotes the health of the corpus luteum, which secretes progesterone following ovulation.

Although testosterone is typically associated with men, women do generate some testosterone, albeit less.

The purposes of testosterone

Preserves Muscle Mass: Assists in maintaining bone and muscle mass.

Libido Support: Encourages arousal of the lust for sex.

Affects Mood and Energy: Has an impact on both general energy levels and mood.

Handling Unbalanced Hormones

Relieving menopausal symptoms and preserving general health depend on controlling hormone imbalances.

Nutrition: Natural hormone balancing can be achieved with a balanced diet high in phytoestrogens, which are present in soy products, flaxseeds, and some legumes. Make sure you're getting enough calcium and vitamin D to maintain healthy bones.

Exercise: Getting regular exercise helps strengthen bones, regulate weight, and elevate mood. Exercises involving weight bearing, such as running, walking, and resistance training, are especially advantageous.

Suitable Sleep Position: Create a consistent sleep schedule. Steer clear of electronics and caffeine right before bed. Reduce night sweats by creating a cool, cozy resting space.

Stress management: Methods like deep breathing exercises, yoga, and meditation can help lower stress and elevate mood.

Healthcare Procedures

Hormone Replacement Therapy (HRT): By substituting the hormones the body no longer makes, HRT can help reduce symptoms. Hormone replacement therapy comes in several forms, such as combined estrogen-progesterone and estrogen-only treatments. Speak with a healthcare professional to decide which course of action is best.

Non-Hormonal Medications: Certain antidepressants and blood pressure medications, as well as some antidepressants, are non-hormonal medications that can help manage symptoms like mood swings and hot flashes for women who cannot take HRT.

Medication for Bone Health: Drugs like selective estrogen receptor modulators (SERMs) and bisphosphonates can help treat and prevent osteoporosis.

Organic Solutions

Supplements with Herbs: Popular herbal remedies like red clover, evening primrose oil, and black cohosh assist some women manage their symptoms. Be sure to speak with your doctor before beginning any supplementation.

Acupuncture: According to some research, acupuncture may be able to reduce mood swings, hot flashes, and other menopausal symptoms.

Mind-Body Techniques: Techniques like mindfulness meditation and tai chi can help lower stress levels, elevate mood, and promote general wellbeing.

Individual Narratives

Personal experiences can offer insightful advice and encouragement. The following two short stories serve as examples of how women handle the hormonal shifts that occur during menopause:

Jane's Nutritional Approach

As Jane, a fifty-year-old teacher, reached menopause, she began to get heat flashes and mood swings. She made the decision to pay closer attention to her food and increased the amount of soy and flaxseeds in her meals. She also started taking a vitamin to help maintain the condition of her bones. Following these dietary adjustments, Jane saw a notable decrease in her symptoms and an increase in her sense of bodily control.

Susan's Workout Schedule

Susan, 48, was having trouble adjusting to menopause and was experiencing anxiety and weight increase. She made the decision to sign up for a local gym and began doing yoga and weightlifting workouts.

She was able to control her weight and her mood thanks to the exercise.

Susan also discovered that attending group classes at the gym had a social component that offered extra emotional support.

It's essential to comprehend how hormones play a part in menopause in order to control symptoms and preserve wellness.

Hormonal shifts can significantly affect a number of facets of life, but they can be successfully navigated with the correct information and techniques.

Hormonal imbalances can be managed in a variety of ways, from lifestyle modifications and pharmacological interventions to natural remedies and personal narratives. You can enter this new stage of life with confidence.

CHAPTER THREE

Nutrition Basics for Menopausal Women

Essential Nutrients for Hormonal Health

A woman's body undergoes major changes throughout menopause, which makes eating a healthy diet even more important. Comprehending the foods that uphold hormonal balance can aid in symptom management and enhance general wellbeing.

Vitamin D and calcium

Bone Health: During menopause, there may be a decrease in bone density due to a drop in estrogen levels, which increases the risk of osteoporosis. Vitamin D and calcium are essential for keeping strong bones.

Sources of Calcium: Dairy foods such as cheese, yogurt, and milk are high in calcium. Almonds, leafy greens, and fortified meals like plant-based milk and orange juice are examples of non-dairy sources.

Sources of Vitamin D: Vitamin D aids in the body's absorption of calcium. While exposure to sunlight is a natural source, diet-related sources include supplements, dairy products with added nutrients, and fatty fish.

magnesium

Magnesium's significance in energy production, neuronal transmission, and muscle function is well-established. Additionally, it helps aid with sleep difficulties that are frequently brought on by menopause.

Sources of Magnesium: Whole grains, nuts, seeds, and leafy green vegetables are good providers of magnesium.

Fatty Acids Omega-3

Heart Health and Inflammation: As the risk of cardiovascular disease rises after menopause, omega-3 fatty acids play a critical role in supporting heart health and reducing inflammation.

Sources of Omega-3s: Rich in omega-3s are fatty fish, such as sardines, mackerel, and salmon. Walnuts, chia seeds, and flaxseeds are examples of plant-based sources.

Phytoestrogens

Hormonal Balance: Plant-based substances called phytoestrogens function similarly to estrogen in the body. Certain menopausal symptoms, such as hot flashes and night sweats, may be lessened by them.

Sources of Phytoestrogens: Legumes, flaxseeds, and soy products (tofu, tempeh, and edamame) are excellent providers of phytoestrogens.

Energy and Mood: The production of energy and cognitive function are dependent on B vitamins, especially B6 and B12. They can aid in reducing menopausal fatigue and mood changes.

Sources of B vitamins include meat, dairy products, eggs, whole grains, and leafy green vegetables.

Vitamin E

Skin and Hair Health: During menopause, skin and hair can become dry and brittle. Vitamin E, an antioxidant, helps maintain healthy skin and hair.

Sources of Vitamin E: Avocados, nuts, seeds, and spinach are high in this nutrient.

Iron

Preventing Anemia: Iron deficiency anemia can result from heavy monthly flow, which some women experience during the perimenopause.

Sources of Iron: High-iron foods include lentils, beans, fish, chicken, red meat, and fortified cereals.

Zinc

Immune System Support: Zinc can aid in the treatment of skin conditions like acne, which some women get as a result of hormone swings.

Sources of Zinc: Dairy products, meat, seafood, legumes, seeds, and nuts are all excellent sources of zinc.

Maintaining general health and controlling menopausal symptoms require a balanced diet. This is how to plan your meals so that you obtain the nutrients you require.

Stress Whole Foods

Nutrient Density: Whole foods, free of processed foods' bad fats and added sugars, are rich in important nutrients. Examples of these foods are fruits, vegetables, whole grains, and lean proteins.

Fruits and Vegetables: To guarantee a range of vitamins, minerals, and antioxidants, aim for a variety of hues. Particularly advantageous foods include cruciferous vegetables, berries, citrus fruits, and leafy greens.

Whole Grains: To improve fiber consumption and support a healthy weight, swap out refined grains for whole grains such as brown rice, quinoa, oats, and whole wheat products.

Lean Proteins: To promote muscle building and general health, use sources including fish, poultry, turkey, beans, lentils, and tofu.

Good Fats

Hormonal Balance: For the body to produce hormones and to function normally, healthy fats are necessary.

Sources of Good Fats: Essential fatty acids and hormone balance are provided by avocados, nuts, seeds, olive oil, and fatty seafood.

Drinking Water

Fluid Balance: Drinking enough water is essential for good health and can help control symptoms such as dry skin and hot flashes.

Water Intake: Try to consume eight glasses or more each day. Adapt according to activity level, weather, and personal requirements.

Hydrating Foods: To help meet hydration needs, include foods high in water, such as cucumbers, melons, oranges, and soups.

Steer clear of processed foods and excessive sugars.

Blood Sugar Stability: Consuming too much sugar can exacerbate menopausal symptoms, cause weight gain, and raise the risk of diabetes.

Limit Sugary Foods: Cut back on sweets, sugar-filled beverages, and high-sugar snacks.

Select Sugars That Are Natural: Choose natural sweeteners sparingly, such as honey or maple syrup.

Practices of Mindful Eating
Listen to Your Body: Mindful eating helps you avoid overindulging and encourage a positive relationship with food by helping you recognize your body's signals of hunger and fullness.

Consume Gradually: Savor your food slowly and pay attention to your body's cues.

Steer clear of distractions: You can better concentrate on the act of eating and identify when you're full by avoiding distractions like TV and smartphones while you're eating.

The Value of Hydration

Staying hydrated is essential for preserving health and controlling menopausal symptoms. Here's why it matters and how to make sure you're drinking enough water.

Advantages of Adequate Hydration

Controls Body Temperature: Staying properly hydrated aids in controlling body temperature, which is especially beneficial for hot flashes and nocturnal sweats.

Promotes Digestion: Water is necessary for a healthy digestive system and can aid in avoiding constipation, which is a typical problem during menopause.

Preserves Skin Health: Adequate hydration helps lessen dryness and increase skin suppleness.

Boosts Energy: Fatigue can result from dehydration. Maintaining fluid intake helps sustain energy levels all day.

Helps with Weight Management: Thirst is sometimes confused with hunger. Avoiding needless snacking can be achieved by drinking enough of water.

Advice on Maintaining Hydration

Carry a Water Bottle: To promote consistent drinking throughout the day, always have a reusable water bottle on you.

Set Reminders: Remind yourself to frequently drink water by using apps or reminders.

Give Your Water Taste: If you find plain water boring, try adding slices of lemon, cucumber, or mint for some natural flavoring.

Keep an eye on your intake: Monitor your water use to make sure you're fulfilling your daily water requirements.

Prior to meals, sip water. Drinking a glass of water before meals can improve digestion and make you feel fuller.

Hydration Without Water

Although water is the ideal beverage for staying hydrated, you can increase your daily fluid intake by consuming other foods and drinks.

Herbal Teas: Without added sugar or caffeine, herbal teas are an excellent way to up your fluid intake.

Soups and broths can be hydrating and nutritious.

Foods High in Water: Include foods high in water in your diet, such as lettuce, cucumbers, strawberries, and watermelon.

Linda's Hydration Experience

Hot flashes and low energy were problems for 52-year-old Linda, a marketing executive, throughout the day. Upon speaking with her physician, she became aware that she was dehydrating. Linda began bringing a water bottle to work and programmed her phone to remind her to drink every hour. She also drank a glass of water before she ate. Linda experienced a decrease in her hot flashes and an increase in her energy levels in a matter of weeks, proving the potent effects of maintaining hydration.

Key tactics for treating menopausal symptoms and preserving general health include knowing the vital nutrients and creating a balanced diet. In this process, hydration is essential since it affects everything from skin health to energy levels. Menopausal women might have greater ease and well-being during this transitional period by emphasizing whole foods, healthy fats, mindful eating practices, and making sure they are getting enough water. Getting on board with these nutrition basics can have a big impact on your daily mood and empower you to face challenges head-on with resilience and confidence.

CHAPTER FOUR

Eating Plans for Weight Loss

Hormonal changes during menopause might impact fat distribution and metabolism, making weight management difficult. Still, following some diet regimens can be beneficial. This chapter will examine the benefits and drawbacks of low-carb, intermittent fasting, and Mediterranean diets, as well as how they can help with weight loss during menopause.

Low-Carb Diets: Pros and Cons

Pros of Low-Carb Diets: Suitable for Losing Weight It has been demonstrated that low-carb diets, such the Atkins diet and the ketogenic diet, are beneficial for weight loss. Weight reduction results from forcing the body to use fat instead of carbohydrates for energy.

Better Blood Sugar Levels: Reducing the amount of carbohydrates you eat can help you better control your blood sugar, which is especially helpful for women who are at risk of type 2 diabetes during menopause.

Decreased Appetite: Diets low in carbohydrates frequently cause people to eat less, which can aid in managing their weight. Since they are more satiating, proteins and fats keep you fuller for longer.

Enhanced Energy: As the body grows more adept at burning fat for fuel, many people who follow a low-carb diet report having more energy and mental clarity.

Cons of Low-Carb Diets

Hard to Maintain: It might be challenging to stick to a low-carb diet over the long haul. They frequently call for drastic dietary adjustments and the removal of many popular foods.

Potential Nutrient Deficiencies: You run the risk of deficient in important nutrients like fiber, vitamins, and minerals if you eliminate or substantially reduce foods high in carbohydrates, such as whole grains, legumes, and fruits.

Potential adverse Effects: When starting a low-carb diet, some people report experiencing adverse effects such headaches, lethargy, and intestinal problems. Often referred to as the "keto flu," these symptoms normally go away in a few days or weeks.

Jane's Low-Carb Experimentation

Jane, a 49-year-old nurse, experienced difficulty gaining weight during menopause. She made the decision to attempt a low-carb diet, eliminating most carbohydrates and putting more of an emphasis on healthy fats and proteins. Jane saw a noticeable reduction in weight and an increase in energy after a few weeks. She did, however, find it difficult to stick to the diet over time and missed her favorite dishes high in carbohydrates.

Jane eventually discovered a balanced strategy that helped her keep the weight off. It included moderate amounts of carbohydrates while still placing a strong emphasis on proteins and fats.

Comprehending Periodic Fasting

Cycling between eating and fasting phases is known as intermittent fasting (IF). The two most popular are the 16/8 approach, which involves fasting for 16 hours and eating within an 8-hour window, and the 5:2 method, which involves five days of regular eating followed by two days of calorie restriction.

The Advantages of Intermittent Fasting

Weight Loss: By lowering total caloric intake and enhancing the body's ability to burn fat, intermittent fasting has been shown to be beneficial for weight loss.

Better Metabolic Health: IF can help during menopause by lowering blood sugar, reducing inflammation, and increasing insulin sensitivity.

Enhanced Autophagy: Autophagy is a process that the body uses to repair damaged cells and grow new ones, which improves general health. It is triggered by fasting periods.

The Difficulties of Intermittent Fasting

Difficult to Begin: With possible side effects like hunger, anger, and weariness, the initial adjustment to fasting periods can be difficult.

Not Suitable for Everyone: IF is not recommended for people with eating disorders or specific medical issues. A healthcare professional must be consulted before beginning any fasting program.

Laura's Experience with Intermittent Fasting

During menopause, 52-year-old Laura, a teacher, battled weight gain and reduced energy. With an aim to practice intermittent fasting (16/8), she made the decision to eat between midday and 8 PM. Although the first week was difficult, she quickly got used to it, saw an increase in her energy, and began to lose weight. Laura liked how IF was easy to use—there was no need to track calories or limit particular meals. She began to feel better and more in charge of her eating patterns over time.

How to Manage Your Weight with the Mediterranean Diet

An outline of the Mediterranean diet

The customary eating patterns of the nations that abut the Mediterranean Sea serve as the foundation for the

Mediterranean diet. Whole meals, good fats, lean proteins, and an abundance of fruits and vegetables are emphasized.

Essential Elements of a Mediterranean Diet

Healthy Fats: The main sources of fat that support heart health and lower inflammation include nuts, seeds, and olive oil.

Fruits and Vegetables: A wide range of vibrant fruits and vegetables offer vital antioxidants, vitamins, and minerals.

Whole Grains: Refined grains should not be used in place of whole grains, such as brown rice, quinoa, and whole wheat products.

Lean Proteins: The primary sources of protein are fish, chicken, beans, and legumes; consumption of red meat should be kept to a minimum.

Moderate Dairy: Cheese and other dairy products should be consumed in moderation.

Red Wine in Moderation: Although it's optional, certain Mediterranean diet regimens call for moderate red wine consumption.

The Mediterranean Diet's advantages

Encourages Weight Loss: The diet's focus on wholesome, high-nutrient meals and good fats can aid in weight reduction and maintenance.

Promotes Heart Health: The heart health advantages of the Mediterranean diet, such as lowered risk of cardiovascular disease, are well-known.

Reduces Inflammation: The foods in this list have anti-inflammatory qualities that can aid in the management of menopausal symptoms and the advancement of general health.

Sustainable and pleasurable: The Mediterranean diet is easy to stick to over the long run because it is adaptable and emphasizes scrumptious, filling foods.

Maria's Triumphant Adoption of the Mediterranean Diet

Maria, a 55-year-old graphic designer, found it difficult to stick to a sustainable diet plan after going through menopause and gaining weight. She made the decision to attempt the Mediterranean diet after learning about it. Maria said it was simple to follow the diet and like the diversity and tastes of the items. She started to lose weight as a result of eating meals high in fish, veggies, and olive oil. Maria adopted a long-term lifestyle shift after noticing changes in her attitude and energy levels.

Mediterranean diet vs. intermittent fasting vs. low-carb

The optimal option will rely on personal tastes, lifestyle, and health requirements. Each of these eating programs has specific advantages and disadvantages. This is a brief analogy:

Low-Carbohydrate Diet:

Advantages: Helps lower hunger, improve blood sugar regulation, and aid in rapid weight loss.

Cons: Difficult to maintain, probable dietary inadequacies, potential adverse reactions.

intermittent fasting:

Advantages: Easy to follow, helps with weight loss, enhances metabolic health, and encourages autophagy.

Cons: Requires consistency, might be difficult at first, and isn't for everyone.

The Mediterranean Diet

Advantages: Encourages weight loss, strengthens heart health, lowers inflammation, and is long-lasting.

Cons: May not lead to rapid weight loss; requires access to a range of fresh meals.

Combining Diets to Get the Best Outcomes

For some women, the easiest way to follow these diets is to combine parts of them. For instance, combining intermittent fasting with the tenets of the Mediterranean diet can yield the advantages of both diets. As an alternative, it may be useful to begin with a low-carb diet for rapid weight loss and then switch to a Mediterranean diet for long-term maintenance.

Useful Advice on Creating a Diet Plan

Start Gradually: Rather of drastically altering your diet all at once, make small adjustments over time. This method raises the possibility of long-term success while assisting your body in adjusting.

Plan Your Meals: Make sure you have the correct foods on hand and steer clear of bad options by planning your meals and snacks.

Keep Yourself Hydrated: Maintaining adequate hydration promotes weight loss and general wellness.

Seek Support: To maintain motivation and get individualized advice, think about working with a nutritionist or joining a support group.

Pay Attention to Your Body: Observe your reactions to various cuisines and eating styles. Based on your body's reactions, modify your diet.

It's a personal journey to select the best food plan for weight loss during menopause. The secret is to choose a sustainable strategy that works for your lifestyle and health objectives, whether that means following the Mediterranean diet, low-carbohydrate diet, or intermittent fasting. Every one of these diets has unique advantages and difficulties, and often the best outcomes come from mixing aspects from other regimens. Recall to plan your meals, remain hydrated, and ask for help when you need it. You may reach your weight loss objectives and manage the hormonal changes associated with menopause with the appropriate approach, which will enhance your overall health and wellbeing.

CHAPTER FIVE

Improving Mood with Nutrition

It can be difficult to manage the emotional ups and downs that come with menopause, but maintaining and enhancing mood can be greatly aided by eating a healthy diet. This chapter looks at foods that raise serotonin levels, the health advantages of omega-3 fatty acids, and how nutrition can help manage stress.

Foods that Elevate Serotonin Levels: An Overview

One neurotransmitter that has a big impact on mood, sleep, and general wellbeing is serotonin. Serotonin, also known as the "feel-good" hormone, is mostly found in the brain, intestines, and blood platelets. Serotonin is involved in mood regulation, anxiety reduction, and happiness; low serotonin levels are associated with depression.

1. Foods High in Tryptophan

The amino acid tryptophan is transformed by the body into serotonin. Including foods high in tryptophan in your diet can help raise serotonin levels.

Chicken and turkey make great sources of tryptophan.
Eggs: Eggs have the ability to enhance serotonin synthesis, particularly when eaten with the yolk.

Cheese: Tryptophan-rich varieties like Swiss and cottage cheese are especially recommended.

Nuts and Seeds: Pumpkin, walnut, sunflower, and almond seeds are all excellent choices.

2. Nutritious Carbohydrates

The availability of tryptophan in the brain can be enhanced by complex carbs, which will raise serotonin levels.

Whole Grains: whole wheat bread, brown rice, and oats.

Starchy Vegetables: corn, squash, and sweet potatoes.

Legumes: Chickpeas, lentils, and beans.

3. Fatty Acids Omega-3

Omega-3 fatty acids have been demonstrated to enhance mood and lessen depressive symptoms, and they are essential for the health of the brain.

Fatty Fish: Omega-3 fatty acids are abundant in salmon, mackerel, and sardines.

Chia and flaxseeds are two great plant-based sources of omega-3 fatty acids.

Another excellent plant-based source of omega-3 fatty acids is walnuts.

4. Foods with fermentation

Gut health is positively correlated with mental health, and fermented foods support gut health. Serotonin synthesis can be increased by a healthy stomach.

Yogurt: Check the label for live, active cultures.

Kefir is a probiotic-rich fermented milk beverage.

Kimchi and sauerkraut are examples of fermented veggies that are good for the gut.

5. Dark Chocolate

Many substances included in dark chocolate, such as antioxidants and tryptophan, have the ability to raise serotonin levels.

Personal Narrative: Susan's Experience Using Foods That Boost Serotonin

Susan, a fifty-year-old educator, experienced melancholy and mood changes during her menopause. She began adding more items high in serotonin to her diet after reading about how nutrition affects mood. She ate eggs and whole-grain bread for breakfast, snacked on nuts and seeds, and twice a week included fatty fish in her meals. Susan's mood and energy levels significantly improved in a matter of weeks, highlighting the potent impact of nutrition on mental health.

Omega-3 Fatty Acids' Function

The importance of Omega-3s

Essential fats that the body is unable to create on its own are omega-3 fatty acids. They are essential for maintaining overall mental health, reducing inflammation, and supporting brain function. Although fish is the main source of omega-3s, they can also be found in some plant sources and supplements.

Omega-3 Fatty Acid Types

EPA and DHA, or eicosapentaenoic acid and docosahexaenoic acid,

Long-chain omega-3 fatty acids, such as EPA and DHA, are present in marine foods including fish and algae. They have been demonstrated to lessen anxiety and depressive symptoms and are very advantageous for brain health.

2. ALA, or alpha-linolenic acid

Plant sources of short-chain omega-3 fatty acids include walnuts, chia seeds, and flaxseeds. Although ALA can be converted by the body into EPA and DHA, the rate of conversion is not very high.

Omega-3s' Advantages for Menopausal Women

1. Improvement of Mood

Numerous studies have demonstrated the potential of omega-3 fatty acids to reduce depressive symptoms and elevate mood. Better emotional regulation may result from their improved neuronal connection and brain function.

2. Mental Ability

In addition to being necessary for preserving cognitive function, omega-3 fatty acids may also assist prevent the aging-related cognitive decline. This is especially crucial during menopause, when some women have trouble focusing and losing their memories.

3. Inflammation Reduction

Because chronic inflammation is connected to a number of health problems, including anxiety and depression, omega-3 fatty acids may help lower it.

Methods for Including Omega-3s in Your Diet

1. Consume Fish That Is Fat.

Include fatty fish in your diet at least twice a week, such as sardines, mackerel, and salmon. These fish have high EPA and DHA content.

2. Include Plant-Based Resources

Incorporate plant-based omega-3 sources into your meals and snacks, such as walnuts, chia seeds, and flaxseeds. Add chia seeds to your smoothies, mix in flaxseeds to your yogurt, or just nibble on some walnuts.

3. Take Supplements Into Account

If you would rather take a plant-based supplement, think about taking an algae-based supplement or fish oil supplement if you find it difficult to obtain enough omega-3s from diet alone. A healthcare professional should always be consulted before beginning any supplement regimen.

Linda's Omega-3 Experience

During menopause, 48-year-old Linda, an accountant, suffered from extreme mood swings and cognitive fog. Her physician advised her to consume more omega-3 fatty acids. Linda started taking a daily fish oil supplement, eating salmon twice a week, and including flaxseeds into her porridge in the morning. After a few months, Linda's mood, mental clarity, and general wellbeing all showed notable gains. This alteration brought to light the significant influence of omega-3s on mental wellness.

Using Diet to Manage Stress

Stress-Relieving Foods

Certain nutrients can strengthen the neurological system and reduce inflammation, which can help the body manage stress more effectively. You can reduce stress and elevate your mood by including these nutrients in your diet.

1. Magnesium

One mineral that is essential for controlling the body's reaction to stress is magnesium. It can enhance the quality of sleep, ease muscle tension, and boost nervous system function.

Leafy green vegetables, legumes, whole grains, nuts, and seeds are some of the sources.

2. B-Complex Vitamin

B vitamins are crucial for preserving mental health, especially B6, B9 (folate), and B12. They aid in the synthesis of dopamine and serotonin as well as energy production and brain function.

Sources: Fish, meat, poultry, eggs, whole grains, and leafy green vegetables.

3. Vitamin D

Depression and mood disorders have been connected to vitamin D deficiency. Making sure you have enough vitamin D in your body might help elevate your mood and lessen depressive symptoms.

Sources: Supplements, fatty fish, sunshine, and fortified dairy products.

4. Antioxidants

Oxidative stress can have a detrimental effect on mental health, but antioxidants help prevent it. In particular, vitamins C and E are crucial for minimizing the harm that stress causes to the body.

Sources: Whole grains, nuts, seeds, and fruits and vegetables.

Avoidable Foods and Drinks

A few foods and beverages have the potential to worsen stress and lower mood. It's critical to restrict your consumption of these things and to be aware of them.

1. Caffeine

Although taking too much coffee can give you a short-term energy boost, it can also raise anxiety, jitters, and interfere with your sleep. Reduce the amount of tea, coffee, and energy drinks you consume.

2. Sugar

An excessive sugar intake might cause mood swings and energy dumps. Reduce your intake of sugary drinks, snacks, and sweets in favor of complete, nutrient-dense foods.

3. Alcohol

While alcohol may initially appear to alleviate stress, it can eventually worsen anxiety and depression and disrupt sleep. When it comes to alcohol drinking, moderation is essential.

1. Make a balanced meal plan

Make sure your meals contain a range of nutrients, such as complex carbohydrates, protein, healthy fats, and an abundance of fruits and vegetables. This equilibrium promotes general health and aids in mood regulation.

2. Maintain Hydration

Drinking enough water is crucial for both physical and emotional well-being. Drink as many glasses of water as possible during the day, and avoid dehydrating drinks like alcohol and coffee.

3. Make Eating Mindful

Eating mindfully entails focusing on your meal, enjoying every bite, and avoiding outside distractions while eating. By doing this, you can lessen tension, facilitate better digestion, and enjoy your food more.

4. Eat Wisely

Stock up on nutritious snacks like fruits, veggies, nuts, and seeds. Steer clear of manufactured snacks that are heavy in sugar and bad fats, as these can have a detrimental effect on your energy and mood.

Karen's Nutritional Adjustments to Reduce Stress

Project manager Karen, 47, experienced extreme stress at work, which caused anxiety and mood swings. She changed a few things after finding out how stress is affected by nutrition. Karen began including more foods high in magnesium, such as almonds and leafy greens, into her meals. In addition, she made sure she had enough sunlight exposure for vitamin D and took a daily supplement of vitamin B complex. Karen also stopped drinking coffee and began to eat mindfully. She saw a noticeable improvement in her general mood and a major decrease in her stress levels within a few months.

Enhancing mood with diet is an effective tactic, especially during menopause when hormone fluctuations might impact mental well-being. You may improve your mood and general well-being by include foods that raise serotonin levels, making sure you're getting enough omega-3 fatty acids, and using your diet to manage stress. Recall that minor dietary adjustments can have a significant impact. Pay attention to your body, choose your meals carefully, and relish the process of achieving greater happiness and mental health.

CHAPTER SIX

Enhancing Sleep Quality

Because of the hormonal changes that impact sleep patterns after menopause, getting good sleep can be especially difficult. This chapter focuses on the critical impact that nutrition can have in improving the quality of your sleep. We'll talk about how to make a diet that is sleep-friendly, the effects of alcohol and caffeine, and foods that help you sleep better.

Foods that Help You Sleep Better

Knowing Your Sleep and Nutrition

There is a strong correlation between sleep and eating. By affecting the release of hormones and neurotransmitters that promote sleep, some meals can aid in the regulation of sleep patterns. Your ability to fall and remain asleep can be significantly improved by include these foods in your diet.

Important Components that Promote Sleep

1. Beta-amylase

The body needs tryptophan, an important amino acid, to make serotonin, a neurotransmitter that controls sleep. Melatonin is the hormone responsible for regulating sleep-wake cycles when serotonin is transformed.

Sources: Dairy products, nuts, seeds, bananas, poultry, and turkey.

2. Calcium

One mineral that is essential for both neurotransmitter modulation and muscle relaxation is magnesium. It can enhance the quality of sleep and aid in nervous system calmdown.

Leafy green vegetables, legumes, whole grains, nuts, and seeds are some of the sources.

3. Calcium

The brain needs calcium in order to utilise tryptophan to produce melatonin. It also aids in controlling muscle contractions, which can interfere with sleep.

Sources: Almonds, broccoli, leafy greens, and dairy products.

4. B6 vitamin

Serotonin and melatonin are produced from tryptophan with the aid of vitamin B6. Sufficient amounts of B6 are essential for the synthesis of these hormones linked to sleep.

Fish, chicken, chickpeas, bananas, and fortified cereals are some of the sources.

1. Almonds

Magnesium is found in abundance in almonds, and this mineral may aid with better sleep. They also supply good fats that promote general health.

2. Kiwi

Vitamins C and K are among the many vitamins and antioxidants found in kiwi fruit. Research has indicated that eating kiwis before bed can increase the quantity and quality of sleep.

3. Cherry Tart Juice

One of the rare natural sources of melatonin is tart cherries. A glass of sour cherry juice before bed will raise melatonin levels and enhance the quality of your sleep.

4. Oily Fish

Fish rich in omega-3 fatty acids and vitamin D include salmon, mackerel, and trout. These nutrients improve the quality of sleep via regulating serotonin.

5. Tea with Chamomile

Apigenin, an antioxidant included in chamomile tea, binds to specific brain receptors that may increase drowsiness and lessen sleeplessness.

Laura's Path to Enhanced Sleep Quality

During her menopause, 52-year-old Laura, a nurse, experienced sleeplessness. Trying to get better sleep, she decided to concentrate on her food. Laura increased the amount of leafy greens and fatty fish in her diet and began snacking on a handful of almonds every evening. Before going to bed, she also drank a cup of chamomile tea. Laura saw a notable increase in her quality of sleep in a matter of weeks, proving the effectiveness of nutrition in addressing sleep-related problems.

The Effects of Alcohol and Caffeine

Coffee and Sleep Disturbances

Well known stimulant caffeine inhibits the effects of the neurotransmitter adenosine, which is known to promote sleep, making it difficult to fall asleep. Making smarter decisions to enhance the quality of your sleep can be aided by knowing how caffeine affects your body.

1. The Caffeine Half-Life

Caffeine's half-life, or how long it takes the body to break down half of the amount ingested, is roughly five to six hours. This implies that taking caffeine in the late afternoon or evening can seriously interfere with your ability to fall asleep.

2. Coffee Sensitivity

Caffeine sensitivity differs from person to person. Some people have slower metabolisms than others, which makes them more vulnerable to the negative effects of caffeine on sleep. It's critical to recognize your individual sensitivity and modify your caffeine use accordingly.

3. Where to Get Coffee

Caffeine can also be present in tea, chocolate, energy drinks, and some pharmaceuticals. You can better control your total consumption by being aware of all possible sources.

Alcohol and the Quality of Sleep

Although alcohol may initially make you feel drowsy, it can seriously disturb your sleep cycle and lower the quality of your sleep.

1. REM Sleep Interrupted

Rapid eye movement (REM) sleep, which is linked to dreaming and memory consolidation, can be disrupted by alcohol. When REM sleep is disturbed, it can cause insomnia at night and weariness the following day.

2. A Rise in Wakefulness at Night

Because alcohol is metabolized by the body during the night, it might lead to repeated awakenings. Sleep that is fragmented and of worse overall quality may arise from this.

3. Sleep and Dehydration

Since alcohol is a diuretic, it can cause dehydration by increasing the output of urine. Dehydration might make you uncomfortable and wake you up at night.

Controlling Alcohol and Caffeine Consumption

Limit your intake of caffeine

Try consuming as little caffeine as possible during the morning. If you're a fan of tea or coffee, choose decaffeinated options in the afternoon and at night.

2. Exercise Caution When consuming alcohol

If you do drink, try to limit your intake and stay away from it right before bed. Alcohol and water consumption together can lessen the effects of dehydration.

3. Pay Attention to Your Responses

Observe your body's reaction to alcohol and coffee. Maintaining a sleep journal might assist you in seeing trends and making the required changes to enhance the quality of your sleep.

The 55-year-old software engineer John found that after consuming a glass of wine before bed and coffee in the afternoon, the quality of his sleep decreased. John made some adjustments after discovering how alcohol and coffee affected his ability to sleep. After lunch, he began drinking decaffeinated coffee and saved his alcohol usage until the early evening. John was able to get deeper, more restful sleep because to these modifications.

Developing a Diet That Promotes Sleep

A Balanced Diet's Role

The vital elements required for general health, including sleep health, are found in a balanced diet. You can make sure you get all the vitamins and minerals you need to support sound sleep by eating a variety of meals.

Timing of Meals and Sleep

1. Consistent mealtimes

Eating meals at regular intervals aids in the internal clock regulation of your body. In order to maintain a regular sleep schedule, try to eat your meals at the same time every day.

2. Skip Large Meals Right Before Bed

Large, heavy meals eaten right before bed can make you uncomfortable and interfere with your sleep. Try to have your final meal two or three hours before bedtime.

3. Small Evening Bites

If you feel like you need a snack before bed, go for something that will help you fall asleep. Healthy foods include yogurt, a tiny banana, and a handful of nuts.

Sleep and Hydration

1. Drink plenty of water

Drinking enough water is important for general health and can affect how well you sleep. Try to stay hydrated during the day, but stay away from excessive amounts right before bed to avoid waking up in the middle of the night.

2. Restrict the use of diuretics

Drinks that cause diuresis, like alcohol and caffeine, should be avoided. These may make it more necessary to urinate at night, which will interfere with your sleep.

Developing a Nighttime Routine that Promotes Sleep

1. Create a Schedule

Your body can be told to wind down and get ready for sleep by following a regular nightly routine. Calming pursuits like reading, having a warm bath, or doing relaxation techniques might be a part of this regimen.

2. Make Your Sleep Environment Ideal

Maintaining a cold, calm, and dark bedroom will help you fall asleep. A comfy mattress and pillows can also have a big impact on how well you sleep.

3. Set Screen Time Limits

It is possible for screen-based blue light exposure to disrupt melatonin production. Aim to spend no more than an hour away from screens before bed. Instead, take part in soothing activities that aid in getting your body and mind ready for sleep.

Emma's Routine and Sleep-Friendly Diet

50-year-old Emma was a graphic artist who suffered from frequent awakenings and poor sleep quality. She altered her diet and nightly routine a few times after looking at techniques to get better sleep. Emma began eating healthy meals on a regular basis, steered clear of large meals right before bed, and included items like kiwis and almonds that help induce sleep. She also created a relaxing bedtime ritual that involved setting a time limit for using screens and reading a book. Emma was able to get more uninterrupted and restful sleep because to these changes.

Improving the quality of sleep with food is an effective strategy, particularly during menopause when sleep disruptions are frequent. You may greatly enhance the quality of your sleep by including foods that aid in better sleep, controlling your consumption of caffeine and alcohol, and developing a diet and routine that are conducive to better sleep. Always remember that minor adjustments might result in big gains. Keep an eye on how your body reacts to various foods and drinks, and adapt as necessary to promote deeper sleep. Savor the trip towards a more peaceful and revitalizing sleep.

CHAPTER SEVEN

Combating Hot Flashes with Diet

One of the most prevalent and annoying menopausal symptoms that many women experience as they move through this life-transitional stage is hot flashes. Fortunately, controlling and lowering the frequency and intensity of hot flashes can be greatly aided by dietary decisions. We will look at foods that can cause hot flashes, foods that can help you calm down, and supplements that might help in this chapter.

Foods to Avoid That Trigger

Recognizing the Causes of Hot Flashes

Abrupt sensations of warmth, hot flashes are frequently accompanied by facial redness and perspiration. A number of things, including specific foods and drinks, can cause them. Detecting and avoiding these triggers can aid in the efficient management of symptoms.

1. Spicy Foods

Foods high in spice are known to increase body temperature and cause hot flashes in a lot of women. Spice-heavy foods and sauces, as well as chili peppers, might make symptoms worse.

Jalapeños, various chili peppers, hot sauces, and spicy curries are among examples.

2. Caffeine

Coffee, tea, chocolate, and some sodas all contain caffeine, which is a stimulant. Hot flashes may result from an increase in body temperature and heart rate.

Energy drinks, chocolate, black tea, green tea, and coffee are some of the sources.

3. Alcohol

Alcohol has the ability to raise body temperature and widen blood vessels, which might result in hot flashes. It also interferes with sleep, which exacerbates general menopausal symptoms.

Sources: Beer, wine, mixed drinks, and other alcoholic drinks.

4. Foods that have been processed

Hot flashes can be brought on by preservatives and chemicals found in highly processed diets. Additionally, they frequently include high levels of sugar and bad fats, both of which can aggravate symptoms and cause weight gain.

Fast food, packaged snacks, sugary cereals, and prepared entrees are a few examples.

Maria, a 48-year-old educator, experienced recurrent episodes of intense flashing. She enjoyed spicy food and coffee, but found that these foods frequently made her problems worse after maintaining a food journal. Maria's quality of life improved when her hot flashes significantly decreased and she began drinking herbal tea instead of spicy foods.

Cooling Foods and Beverages

Foods That Aid in Temperature Regulation

Cooling foods help your body naturally regulate temperature, which can help manage hot flashes. These foods are frequently nutrient-dense and hydrated, supporting general wellness.

1. Vegetables and Fruits

Because they contain a lot of water, fruits and vegetables can help you stay hydrated, which is important for controlling body temperature.

Leafy greens, strawberries, watermelon, and cucumbers are a few examples.

2. Products Made of Soy

Phytoestrogens are plant-based substances found in soy that function similarly to estrogen in the body. These can lessen the frequency of hot flashes and help balance hormone levels.

Sources: Edamame, tempeh, tofu, and soy milk.

3. Flaxseeds

Lignans are a different kind of phytoestrogen that are abundant in flaxseed. They also include omega-3 fatty acids, which are good for inflammation and the heart.

Use: Include ground flaxseeds in salads, yoghurt, and smoothies.

4. Fish from Cold Water

Omega-3 fatty acids, which are abundant in fish like sardines, mackerel, and salmon, might help lower inflammation and enhance general health, which may lessen hot flash symptoms.

Sardines, trout, mackerel, and salmon are a few examples.

Hydrating Beverages

It's essential to drink enough of water to control heat flashes. Hot flashes can be less intense and body temperature can be maintained by drinking lots of water and other hydrating drinks.

1. Water

The greatest choice for staying hydrated is plain water. Try to get eight glasses or more if you live in a hot area or are an active person each day.

2. Herbal Teas

Herbal teas can be calming and hydrating, especially the ones that have cooling qualities. For example, peppermint tea is well-known for its cooling properties.

3. Water from coconuts

A natural electrolyte beverage that might help you stay hydrated and replace minerals lost via perspiration is coconut water.

Susan's Rehydrating Diet

Susan, an artist who was 55 years old, was experiencing intense hot flashes. She started adding more cold foods to her diet, such cucumbers, melons, and soy products, after speaking with a dietitian. She also switched to peppermint tea in place of her afternoon coffee. Susan was able to better control her hot flashes and concentrate on her artwork as a result of these adjustments.

Extras to Help with Hot Flashes

Natural Supplements to Take into Account
Taking certain supplements can help control hot flashes in addition to dietary adjustments. These dietary supplements, which have long been used to promote women's health, are frequently made from plants.

1. Cohosh Black

The herb black cohosh has long been used to alleviate hot flashes and other menopausal symptoms. It is thought to have estrogen-like properties that can aid with hormone balance.

Usage: Available in liquid extract, tablet, and capsule form.

2. The Red Clover

Isoflavones, a kind of phytoestrogen found in red clover, may help lessen the frequency and intensity of hot flashes.

Usage: Teas, pills, and capsules are available.

3. Evening Primrose Oil

Gamma-linolenic acid (GLA), an abundant fatty acid found in evening primrose oil, has anti-inflammatory and anti-hot flash properties.

Use: Capsules are available.

4. Fatty Acids Omega-3

Hot flashes may be less frequent with the use of omega-3 supplements, such as flaxseed or fish oil, which can also help lower inflammation and enhance general health.

Usage: Both liquid and pill versions are available.

It is crucial to speak with a healthcare professional when selecting supplements to make sure they are secure and suitable for your particular requirements. Expert advice is essential because supplements may interfere with drugs and other medical issues.

Linda's Triumph with Supplements

50-year-old Linda was a nurse who frequently had heat flashes that interfered with her day-to-day activities. She made the decision to try black cohosh and omega-3 supplements after reading up on natural therapies. After starting these supplements with her doctor's consent, Linda saw a major decrease in the frequency and intensity of her hot flashes, which improved her performance at work.

Combining Nutrition with Supplements

Dietary adjustments along with the right supplements can offer a complete solution for hot flash control. The following advice can help you successfully incorporate these strategies:

1. Maintain a Food and Symptom Record

Keeping a food and mood journal might be useful in determining triggers and practical solutions. Keep track of any supplements you consume and how they affect your symptoms.

2. Maintain consistency

When it comes to dietary adjustments and supplementation, consistency is essential. Over the course of many weeks, observe your development and allow your body time to adjust.

3. Pay Attention to Your Body

Observe how your body reacts to various diets and substances. Everybody's menopausal experience is different, so what works for one woman might not work for another.

4. Get Expert Counsel

Speaking with a dietitian or healthcare professional will guarantee that your strategy is secure and efficient while also offering tailored advice.

Menopause hot flashes can be difficult to manage, but with the correct vitamins and diet adjustments, they can be greatly reduced. You can lessen the frequency and severity of hot flashes and enhance your general quality of life by staying away from trigger foods, embracing cool meals and beverages, and taking natural supplements sparingly.

Keep in mind that each woman's experience with menopause is different, so it could take some time to figure out what suits you the best. Remain persistent and patient, and don't be afraid to ask medical professionals for help. You can get through this stage of life with greater ease and assurance if you take the appropriate strategy.

CHAPTER EIGHT

Maintaining Bone Health

It becomes more crucial for women to preserve their bone health when they go through menopause. Osteoporosis and fractures are more likely as a result of decreased bone density brought on by a drop in estrogen levels. This chapter will cover nutrients that promote bone density, the critical roles played by calcium and vitamin D, and lifestyle choices that help maintain strong bones.

Consumption of Calcium and Vitamin D

The Value of Calcium

The element calcium is essential for keeping bones strong and dense. The body's capacity to hold calcium diminishes throughout menopause, so it's critical to make sure you're getting enough of it. In addition to being essential for healthy bones, calcium is also involved in blood clotting, neuron transmission, and muscle contraction.

Recommended Daily Consumption:

Ages 19 to 50 for women: 1,000 mg daily

Women 51 years of age and above: 1,200 mg daily

Best Sources of Calcium

Including foods high in calcium in your diet is the best approach to ensure that you get the recommended amount each day.

1. Dairy Products

One of the best sources of calcium is dairy products. They also include a lot of protein, which is good for the whole body.

Examples include cheese, yogurt, and milk

2. Green Leafy Vegetables

For people who choose a plant-based diet or are lactose intolerant, leafy greens are a great plant-based source of calcium.

Examples: collard greens, spinach, and kale

3. Fortified Foods

Calcium is added to a lot of meals, which makes it simpler to get the daily amount you require.

Examples include fortified cereals, plant-based milks (almond, soy, and rice), and fortified orange juice.

4. Fish with Edible Bones

Some fish, particularly those with bones that can be eaten, are a good source of calcium.

For instance, canned salmon and sardines

Vitamin D's Role

For the body to absorb calcium, vitamin D is essential. The body cannot absorb the calcium required to sustain bone health if it does not receive enough vitamin D.

Recommended Daily Consumption:
600 IU (International Units) per day for women aged 19 to 70

Women seventy-one and older: 800 IU daily

Top Vitamin D Sources: 1. Sunlight

When the body is exposed to sunshine, vitamin D is synthesized. A few times a week, spending 10 to 30 minutes in the sun can help maintain appropriate levels.

One of the best dietary sources of vitamin D is fatty fish.

Examples: tuna, mackerel, and salmon

3. Fortified Foods

Like calcium, many foods are fortified with vitamin D.

For instance, cereals, orange juice, and fortified milk

4. Supplements

Supplements might be a useful choice for people who struggle to obtain adequate vitamin D from their food and from sunshine. See a doctor before beginning any new supplementation regimen.

Lisa's Vitamin D and Calcium Regimen

Following menopause, 52-year-old Lisa, an accountant, started to lose bone density. Her physician advised her to take more calcium and vitamin D. Lisa began taking a daily vitamin D supplement, increasing her intake of leafy greens in her diet, and drinking fortified plant-based milk. Her bone density increased in less than a year, and she began to feel more assured about her general health.

Foods to Help Maintain Bone Density

Rich in Nutrients Foods for Healthy Bones

Apart from calcium and vitamin D, several other nutrients are crucial for preserving bone density. Including a range of foods high in nutrients can help maintain bone health overall.

1. Magnesium

Magnesium facilitates the active form of vitamin D, which helps the body absorb calcium. It has a direct role in the development of bones as well.

Sources: Whole grains (quinoa, brown rice), nuts (almonds, cashews), and seeds (pumpkin, chia).

2. Vitamin K

Because it aids in the synthesis of the proteins required for bone development, vitamin K is crucial for maintaining healthy bones

Sources: Brussels sprouts, broccoli, and leafy greens (kale, spinach).

3. Protein

Consuming enough protein is essential for maintaining and repairing bones. It's crucial to balance your protein intake with adequate calcium, though.

Sources: Fish, eggs, beans, dairy products, and lean meats

4. Fatty Acids Omega-3

Because of their anti-inflammatory qualities, omega-3 fatty acids may be able to slow down bone loss.

Sources: walnuts, chia seeds, flaxseeds, and fatty fish (mackerel, salmon).

Sarah's Diet for Strong Bones

Following a scare with low bone density, 55-year-old Sarah, a teacher, concentrated on enhancing her bone health. She began adding a range of foods, including nuts, seeds, fatty fish, and leafy greens, that assist bone structure to her diet. Sarah also started blending plant-based milk into smoothies, incorporating chia seeds for an additional nutritional punch. Her bone density tests improved over time, and she experienced an increase in energy and general health.

Ways of Living for Strong Bones

Physical Activity and Bone Health

The greatest strategy to preserve and increase bone density is to engage in regular physical exercise. Strength training and weightlifting are especially advantageous.

1. Weight-Bearing Exercises

Exercises involving weight bearing require you to defy gravity, which preserves and increases bone density.

Walking, running, hiking, dancing, and stair climbing are a few examples.

2. Exercise for Strength

Muscle mass is increased by strength training activities, supporting and safeguarding bones. By promoting the growth of new bone, it also raises bone density.

Examples include bodyweight exercises (squats, push-ups), resistance band exercises, and weightlifting.

3. Exercises for Flexibility and Balance

Enhancing flexibility and balance can assist avoid falls, which lowers the chance of fractures.

Suggestions: Pilates, Tai Chi, and Yoga

Lifestyle Selections for Healthy Bones

Developing a healthy lifestyle might also help you have stronger bones.

1. Avoid Smoking

Smoking is bad for the health of your bones. It makes it harder for the body to absorb calcium and decreases blood flow to the bones.

2. Limit Your Alcohol Consumption

Drinking too much alcohol can cause bone loss and raise the risk of fractures. It's advisable to keep alcohol consumption in check.

3. Continue to Eat a Healthy Weight

While being overweight can put extra strain on bones and joints, being underweight can raise the risk of bone loss and fractures. Achieve a healthy weight by eating a balanced diet and doing frequent exercise.

4. Keep an eye on bone health

Frequent DEXA scans, or bone density examinations, can monitor bone health and identify any problems early. This makes it possible for prompt management and action.

Nancy's Changes in Exercise and Lifestyle

Nancy, a 60-year-old librarian, was identified as having osteopenia, a disorder characterized by reduced bone density. Nancy began a weight-bearing and strength-training regimen that included walking, weightlifting, and yoga in order to strengthen her bones. She also cut back on her alcohol use and stopped smoking.

Her bone density increased with time, and she experienced increased strength and balance in her day-to-day activities.

Preventing osteoporosis and fractures after menopause requires maintaining bone health. Women may strengthen their bones and enhance their general health by making sure they consume enough calcium and vitamin D, including a range of foods that support bone health, and leading healthy lifestyles.

 Important elements of a bone-healthy lifestyle include staying away from tobacco, drinking in moderation, exercising regularly, and maintaining a healthy weight.

Recall that every woman's menopausal experience is different. It's critical to determine what suits you best and implement small, long-lasting adjustments.

You can have strong, healthy bones and a higher standard of living both during and after menopause if you take the appropriate measures.

CHAPTER NINE

Heart Health During Menopause

It becomes more crucial for women to preserve their heart health when they go through menopause. Adopting heart-healthy practices is crucial since hormonal fluctuations can have an impact on cardiovascular health. This chapter will cover heart-healthy diets, the function of lipids and cholesterol, and dietary strategies for reducing inflammation.

Plans for Heart-Healthy Eating

Mediterranean Diet

The heart health benefits of the Mediterranean diet are well known. Whole foods, healthy fats, and plant-based ingredients are the mainstays of this diet.

Fruits and vegetables: Rich in fiber and antioxidants that promote heart health.

Whole Grains: Offer vital nutrients and support normal blood glucose levels.

Good Fats: Avocados and olive oil are great providers of monounsaturated fats, which are heart-healthy.

Lean Proteins: Omega-3 fatty acids, which promote cardiovascular health, are found in fish, particularly fatty fishlike salmon and mackerel.

Nuts and seeds: Provide a fantastic supply of protein and beneficial fats.

Legumes: Chickpeas, lentils, and beans are rich sources of protein and fiber.

The DASH Diet

A prevalent worry during menopause, high blood pressure is intended to be combated with the Dietary Approaches to Stop Hypertension (DASH) diet.

Important Elements:

Low sodium: Promotes heart health and lowers blood pressure.

Vegetables and Fruits in Plenty: Rich in potassium, which helps regulate salt levels.

Whole Grains: Offer vital minerals and fiber.

Lean Proteins: Places special emphasis on fish, poultry, and plant-based proteins.

Low-Fat Dairy: Vitamin D and calcium sources.

Plant-Based Diet

By cutting back on saturated fats and upping fiber and antioxidant intake, a plant-based diet can dramatically enhance heart health.

Fruits and vegetables: Rich in antioxidants and fiber.

Whole Grains: Packed in fiber and nutrients.

Legumes: Offer fiber and protein.

Nuts and seeds are good sources of protein and good fats.

Plant-based proteins include seitan, tempeh, and tofu.

Karen's Path to Heart Health

As she approached menopause, 52-year-old teacher Karen noticed an increase in her cholesterol. Changing to a Mediterranean diet was advised by her doctor. Karen began to include more whole grains, seafood, fruits, and vegetables in her meals. She also started eating more nuts and seeds and switched from butter to olive oil. Karen experienced an improvement in her cholesterol readings and general health and energy levels within a span of six months.

The Functions of Fats and Cholesterol

Knowing About Cholesterol

One kind of fat that can be present in blood is cholesterol. A high cholesterol diet can cause heart disease even though the body need some cholesterol to operate properly.

various forms of cholesterol

High levels of low-density lipoprotein (LDL), sometimes referred to as "bad" cholesterol, can cause plaque to accumulate in arteries.

High-Density Lipoprotein (HDL): Often referred to as "good" cholesterol, it aids in the elimination of LDL from the blood.

Menopause's Effect on Cholesterol Levels

Heart disease risk can be increased by hormonal changes that occur during menopause, which can result in a decrease in HDL and an increase in LDL.

Good Fats versus Bad Fats

Good Fats:

Avocados, certain nuts, and olive oil are good sources of monounsaturated fats. Lowering LDL levels can be aided by these lipids.

Walnuts, flaxseeds, and fatty fish are good sources of polyunsaturated fats. Omega-3 and omega-6 fatty acids, which promote heart health, are among these lipids.

Unhealthy fats

Red meat, butter, and full-fat dairy products are sources of saturated fats. LDL levels may rise due to these lipids.

Trans fats are present in a lot of processed foods. These lipids have the ability to decrease HDL and increase LDL.

Maria's Control of Her Cholesterol

After going through menopause, Maria, a 55-year-old accountant, was diagnosed with elevated LDL cholesterol. Her physician advised her to consume more healthy fats and less saturated fat. Maria began incorporating more fatty fish into her diet, cooking with olive oil, and nibbling on almonds. Her total heart health improved as her HDL levels rose and her LDL levels fell over time.

Dietary Approaches to Lower Inflammation

Avoiding Inflammatory Foods

There is a connection between an elevated risk of heart disease and inflammation in the body, which can be caused by specific diets.

Foods to Steer Clear of:

Processed foods: Frequently excessive in sugar, salt, and trans fats.

Sugary Drinks: sodas and teas with added sugar.

Refined carbohydrates include processed carbohydrates such as white bread and pastries.

Red Meat: Specifically, processed meats such as sausage and bacon.

Anti-Inflammatory Diets

You can lower inflammation and promote heart health by include anti-inflammatory items in your diet.

Foods to Add:

Fruits and vegetables: High in fiber and antioxidants.

Omega-3 fatty acids are abundant in fatty fish.

Whole Grains: These include brown rice, quinoa, and oats.

Nuts and seeds: Offer antioxidants and good fats.

Herbs and Spices: Garlic, ginger, and turmeric, for example.

Antioxidants' Function

The body can develop inflammation and heart disease as a result of oxidative stress, which antioxidants help prevent. Antioxidant-rich foods include dark chocolate, green tea, and berries.

Anne's Diet of Anti-Inflammation

During menopause, Anne, a 58-year-old nurse, battled inflammation and elevated blood pressure. She chose to concentrate on eating a diet low in inflammation. Anne began to include nuts and fatty fish in her meals, as well as more fruits, veggies, and nutritious grains. She started consuming green tea and cooked with ginger and turmeric. Anne saw a decrease in inflammation and an improvement in her heart's general condition over time.

A vital component of general health is heart health, particularly during menopause. Women can dramatically enhance their cardiovascular health by embracing heart-healthy eating plans, comprehending the importance of fats and cholesterol, and lowering inflammation through nutrition.

A healthy heart can be maintained by avoiding inflammatory diets, emphasizing healthy fats, and incorporating a variety of nutrient-dense foods. Monitoring cholesterol levels and scheduling routine examinations are also critical for maintaining heart health throughout menopause. A happier and more satisfying life might result from striking the correct balance between dietary adjustments and lifestyle modifications, as every woman's menopausal journey is different.

CHAPTER TEN

Boosting Energy Levels

A woman's body may undergo several changes during menopause, one of which is a notable variation in energy levels. During this trimester, a lot of women report feeling tired and generally lacking in energy. This chapter covers diet, lifestyle modifications, and healthy eating practices as ways to increase energy levels.

Foods High in Nutrients for Energy

Whole Grains

Complex carbohydrates can be found in abundance in whole grains such as quinoa, brown rice, oats, and whole wheat. They help to sustain blood glucose levels throughout the day by delivering a consistent flow of the energy-boosting chemical. Additionally high in fiber, whole grains promote better digestion and prolonged feelings of fullness.

As example:

Oatmeal: Have a cup of oatmeal with nuts and fruits on top to start your day.

Quinoa Salad: For a wholesome meal, mix quinoa with beans, veggies, and a mild dressing.

Lean Proteins

Proteins are necessary for both building and repairing muscle, as well as for sustaining steady energy levels. Lean protein options include fish, poultry, tofu, lentils, and chicken. These proteins give you the essential amino acids without any extra lipids that can make you move more slowly.

As example:

Serve the grilled chicken over brown rice and a side of steamed veggies.

A satisfying and substantial choice that is high in fiber and protein is lentil soup.

Vegetables and Fruits

Fruits and vegetables are a great source of antioxidants, vitamins, and minerals that improve general health and energy levels. To make sure your diet is providing you with a wide range of nutrients, include a diversity of colors in it.

As an example:

Berries: High in vitamin C and antioxidants.

Leafy Greens: Swiss chard, spinach, and kale are great providers of magnesium and iron.

Nutrient-dense foods like avocados, almonds, seeds, and olive oil are high in healthy fats that offer sustained energy. They can enhance mood and cognitive performance and are also essential for maintaining the health of the brain.

As an example:

Avocado Toast: For a wholesome breakfast, spread mashed avocado on whole-grain toast.

Nuts and Seeds: For an instant energy boost, keep a combination of almonds, walnuts, and sunflower seeds on hand.

Hydration

Maintaining fluid intake is essential for sustaining energy levels. Fatigue and a decline in cognitive function can result from even slight dehydration. Drink eight glasses of water or more each day, and make sure your diet includes foods high in water content, such as oranges, cucumbers, and watermelon.

Tips:

Infused Water: To give your water a cool touch, add slices of cucumber, lemon, or berries.

Herbal Teas: To stay hydrated and enjoy a relaxing beverage, choose herbal teas without caffeine.

Preventing Energy Dips

Properly Balanced Meals

Maintaining steady energy levels can be achieved by eating meals that are well-balanced and contain a variety of carbs, proteins, and fats. Meals heavy in simple carbs and refined sugars should be avoided because they can quickly raise blood sugar levels and then sharply lower them, leaving you feeling lethargic.

Example of a Menu:

Greek yogurt for breakfast, topped with fresh berries and honey drizzled over.

Lunch consists of mixed vegetables on the side and grilled salmon over quinoa.

Dinner is brown rice and stir-fried tofu with veggies.

Snacks to Maintain Energy

Consuming nutritious snacks might help you stay energized in between meals. Select snacks that will keep you full and energized by combining fiber, protein, and healthy fats.

As an example:

Apple slices with almond butter: a good source of fiber, healthy fats, and natural sugars.

Hummus with Vegetables: Crispy veggies dipped in hummus, which is high in protein.

Managing Caffeine Intake

Although an over reliance on coffee can result in crashes later in the day, it can offer a brief energy boost. Instead of using caffeine during the day, try consuming healthier beverages like matcha or green tea, which offer a more gradual and long-lasting energy boost.

Sarah's Transformation in Energy

Sarah, a 49-year-old marketing executive, had lulls in her energy during the day. She changed her diet to incorporate more whole grains, lean proteins, and healthy fats after speaking with a nutritionist. She also cut back on her afternoon coffee use and began bringing nutritious snacks to work. Sarah's energy and general well-being significantly improved in a matter of weeks.

The Value of Regular Meals

Breakfast: The Most Vital Meal of the Day

A healthy breakfast can influence your energy levels throughout the day. Missing breakfast increases the risk of overindulging later in the day and lowers energy levels.

Ideas for Breakfast:

Blend spinach, frozen berries, bananas, and a speck of protein powder in a smoothie bowl. Sprinkle chia seeds and granola over top.

Egg Muffins: For a high-protein, premade breakfast, bake eggs with diced vegetables in muffin pans.

Midday Snacks

It's essential to have a nutritious lunch if you want to stay energetic throughout afternoon. Steer clear of fatty, heavy foods that can cause you to feel lethargic.

Ideas for Lunch:

Serve this quick and simple stir-fried chicken and vegetables over quinoa or brown rice.

Mediterranean salad: feta cheese, cherry tomatoes, cucumbers, olives, and chickpeas mixed with mixed greens and dressed with lemon juice and olive oil.

Dinner will be balanced and light.

A light, well-balanced meal at the end of the day can help you avoid overindulging and encourage better sleep. Make sure to incorporate nutritious grains, lean protein, and a variety of vegetables.

Ideas for Dinner:

Serve baked salmon with asparagus and sweet potatoes.

Chickpeas, tomatoes, and spinach are combined to make a vegetable curry that is eaten over brown rice.

Continual Meal Routine

Keeping a regular meal schedule reduces the risk of energy dips and helps maintain stable blood sugar levels. Eat meals at regular intervals throughout the day, and feel free to add in little, wholesome snacks as needed.

Jack's Constant Energy

Due to his hectic schedule, 53-year-old Jack, an engineer, frequently skipped meals and depended on coffee to get him through the day.

Following a string of low energy episodes, Jack made the decision to adopt a more regimented eating schedule. He started having regular, well-balanced meals and added nutritious snacks. His energy levels were maintained by the diet adjustment, which also increased his focus and output at work.

Making thoughtful food and meal planning decisions is essential to boosting energy throughout menopause. Including foods high in nutrients, eating a balanced diet to prevent energy dips, and sticking to a regular meal schedule are all important ways to stay energized. Every woman's experience with menopause is different, and achieving a healthy balance between dietary adjustments and lifestyle modifications can result in a more active and satisfying existence.

You can support your body's requirements throughout this transition time by making informed decisions by knowing how different foods affect your energy levels. Recall that even minor adjustments to your food and eating routine can have a big impact on your daily mood.

Thus, accept the adventure while concentrating on giving your body what it needs and increasing your vitality naturally.

CHAPTER ELEVEN

Managing Menopausal Symptoms with Herbs and Supplements

Numerous symptoms associated with menopause can seriously lower a woman's quality of life. Many women look for natural alternatives to medicinal therapies in order to control their symptoms. Popular herbal therapies, important vitamins and minerals for menopausal health, and concerns about the efficacy and safety of supplements are all covered in this chapter. With this knowledge, women can make wise decisions to enhance their menopausal health.

Common Herbal Treatments

Black Cohosh

Well-studied black cohosh is well-known for its ability to reduce menopausal symptoms, including hot flashes and night sweats. Black cohosh is a plant whose roots belong to the buttercup family. Native Americans have long utilized it to treat a variety of illnesses.

How Works:

It is thought that black cohosh affects serotonin receptors, which aids in controlling mood and body temperature. Further research is necessary to confirm the moderate estrogenic effects shown by several investigations.

Usage and Dosage:

The usual dosages are between 20 and 40 mg daily. It comes in a number of forms, such as liquid extracts, tablets, and capsules. Generally speaking, black cohosh should only be used for brief periods of time—up to six months.

Red Clover

Phytoestrogens are plant-based substances found in red clover that function similarly to estrogen in the body.

When natural estrogen levels drop throughout menopause, this may be helpful.

Benefits:

Red clover may enhance cardiovascular health, lessen hot flashes, and increase bone density. Additionally, according to some research, it could lessen mood swings and other emotional problems.

Usage and Dosage:

Red clover supplements are available as tablets, capsules, and teas, among other forms. 40 to 80 milligrams of isoflavones per day is the usual dosage.

Dong Quai

Chinese traditional medicine uses dong quai, sometimes referred to as "female ginseng," to address ailments specific to women's health. Dong quai formulations are often used in conjunction with other herbs to help balance hormones and relieve menopausal symptoms.

Night sweats, vaginal dryness, and hot flashes may all be alleviated by dong quai. It also lessens the chance of osteoporosis and increases blood circulation.

Usage and Dosage:

Most people take dong quai as a tea, tablet, or capsule. A daily dosage of 500–1,000 mg is typical. It should be used cautiously because it might interfere with drugs that thin the blood.

Evening Primrose Oil

Gamma-linolenic acid (GLA), an omega-6 fatty acid with anti-inflammatory qualities, is abundant in evening primrose oil. It is frequently used to reduce mood swings and breast pain, two common menopausal symptoms.

Advantages:

Evening primrose oil may help balance mood, lessen hot flashes, and enhance skin health. Additionally, it can help with various inflammatory disorders and joint pain.

Usage and Dosage:

500–1,000 mg of evening primrose oil should be taken daily on average. Both liquid and pill versions are available.

Sage

Sage is a typical culinary herb with medical benefits for menopausal women. Sage is well known for its capacity to lessen excessive perspiration and hot flashes, making it a useful natural medicine.

Benefits:

Compounds in sage affect the central nervous system to control body temperature and sweating. It also possesses anti-inflammatory and antioxidant qualities.

You can consume sage as a tea, tincture, or supplement. For the purpose of easing menopausal symptoms, 300–600 mg of dried sage leaf should be taken daily.

Valerian Root

Because of its well-known calming qualities, Valerian root is frequently used to encourage sleep and lessen anxiety. It can be especially helpful for menopausal women in controlling their stress and sleeplessness.

Advantages:

Valerian root eases anxiety, shortens the time it takes to fall asleep, and enhances the quality of sleep. Because it encourages relaxation, it might also aid with hot flashes and nocturnal sweats.

Usage and Dosage:

There are drinks, pills, and capsules made from Valerian root. 300–600 milligrams administered 30–2 hours prior to bedtime is the usual dosage.

Minerals and Vitamins for Menopause-Related Health

Vitamin D and calcium

Women who go through menopause are more susceptible to osteoporosis and bone fractures because of the decrease in estrogen levels. Vitamin D and calcium are necessary to keep bones healthy.

Calcium: 1,200 mg of calcium should be consumed daily by women over 50, either through food or supplements. Dairy products, fortified meals, and leafy green vegetables are good dietary sources of calcium.

Vitamin D:

Vitamin D is essential for healthy bones and aids in the body's absorption of calcium. For women over 50, a daily intake of 600–800 international units (IU) is advised. Good sources of vitamin D include foods enriched with nutrients, fatty fish, and sun exposure.

magnesium

Magnesium is necessary for bone health, blood sugar regulation, muscle and neuron function, and more than 300 metabolic processes in the body.

Advantages:

Magnesium has been shown to help lower the incidence of osteoporosis, enhance sleep, and lessen depressive and anxious feelings. It also contributes to blood pressure regulation and heart health maintenance.

Usage and Dosage:

For women over 50, 320 mg of magnesium should be consumed daily. Nuts, seeds, whole grains, and leafy green vegetables are foods high in magnesium. There are also other kinds of magnesium supplements, like magnesium oxide and citrate.

B vitamins

B vitamins are necessary for the synthesis of energy, proper brain function, and mood modulation. In particular, B6, B12, and folic acid are vital.

B6:

The production of neurotransmitters that control mood and sleep is aided by vitamin B6. Additionally, it can lessen anxiety and depressive symptoms.

B12:

Red blood cell formation and nerve function depend on vitamin B12. Both energy levels and cognitive performance may be enhanced by it.

Folic acid is necessary for cell division and growth and aids in the production and repair of DNA.

Usage and Dosage:

It is advised to consume 1.5 milligrams of vitamin B6, 2.4 micrograms of vitamin B12, and 400 micrograms of folic acid every day. Legumes, leafy green vegetables, fortified cereals, and animal products all contain these vitamins.

Vitamin E

Antioxidants like vitamin E aid in preventing cell damage. Its ability to lessen hot flashes and other menopausal symptoms has been researched.

Advantages:

Vitamin E may strengthen the immune system, enhance skin health, and lessen the frequency and intensity of hot flashes.

Usage and Dosage:

For women over 50, 15 mg of vitamin E per day is the recommended dose. Nuts, seeds, vegetable oils, and leafy green vegetables are good providers of vitamin E.

The Security and Performance of Add-ons

Understanding Supplement Labels

It's critical to thoroughly read labels and comprehend what you're consuming when selecting supplements. Seek for supplements that have undergone quality and purity testing from independent agencies.

Important Label Details:

The particular nutrients or botanicals that make up the supplement's active ingredients.

Information about Dosage: The quantity of every component used in a serving.

Other Ingredients: Any other parts, including binders or fillers.

Expiration date: Verifies the effectiveness of the product.

Advising Medical Professionals

See a healthcare professional before beginning any new supplement regimen, particularly if you are taking medication or have pre-existing health conditions. Certain health issues may worsen or certain supplements may interfere with drugs.

Role of Healthcare Provider:

Personalized Advice: Specific suggestions made in light of your medical background and present circumstances.

Medication Interactions: Determine whether your present medications may interact with one another.

Monitoring is keeping an eye on your development and adjusting as necessary.

Maria's Experience Using Herbal Treatments

Maria, a 52-year-old educator, went through the early stages of menopause with severe hot flashes and nocturnal sweats. Having had little luck with over-the-counter drugs, she turned her attention to herbal therapies. Maria began taking supplements including red clover and black cohosh under the advice of a naturopathic physician. She saw a noticeable decrease in the frequency and intensity of her hot flashes within a few weeks. Maria's experience serves as a reminder of the possible advantages of using herbal treatments sensibly and under a doctor's supervision.

Possible adverse effects

Herbs and supplements have the potential to cause negative effects, even as they can provide comfort. It's critical to keep an eye on how your body reacts and to stop using the product if you have any negative side effects, such as headaches, allergic responses, or gastrointestinal distress.

Typical Adverse Reactions:

Problems with the stomach: cramps, diarrhea, or nausea.

Allergic Reactions: Skin irritation, swelling, or itching.

Mild to moderate headaches are experienced.

Select premium supplements from reliable manufacturers. Supplements of poor quality could have impurities or the wrong amounts of active components. Seek for products that independent organizations have evaluated.

Selecting High-Quality Supplements:

Third-Party Testing: Goods having their purity and quality confirmed by impartial labs.

Reputable Brands: Businesses with favorable evaluations and ethical production methods.

Clear Labels: Information regarding substances and dosages that is transparent.

Herbs and vitamins can be a useful and natural way to manage menopausal symptoms. Women can make decisions that will enhance their quality of life during menopause by being aware of the advantages and disadvantages of common herbal therapies, as well as the importance of vitamins and minerals. To guarantee safety and effectiveness, always get advice from a healthcare professional before beginning a new supplement regimen.

CHAPTER TWELVE

Creating a Sustainable Healthy Living Plan

There is more to managing menopausal symptoms than just treating them right away. Developing a long-term, healthy lifestyle plan is essential to overall wellbeing. This chapter focuses on creating long-term health goals, integrating mindfulness and stress management practices, and balancing diet and exercise. Through menopause and beyond, women can sustain a healthy and well-balanced lifestyle by adopting these strategies.

Blending Exercise and Nutrition Together

The Value of Well-Balanced Diet

Maintaining general health and controlling menopausal symptoms require a balanced diet. Foods high in nutrients supply the vitamins and minerals required for bone health, hormone balance, and energy production.

Important Elements of a Well-Blended Diet:

Rich in vitamins, minerals, and antioxidants are fruits and vegetables. To guarantee a diversity of nutrients, aim for a variety of colors.

Lean Proteins: Vital for the upkeep and repair of muscles. Add sources include poultry, fish, beans, and nuts.

Whole Grains: Offer fiber and long-lasting energy. Make choices such as whole-wheat bread, brown rice, and quinoa.

Good Fats: Essential for hormone production and brain function. Add fatty seafood, avocados, and olive oil.

Advantages of Frequent Exercise

Engaging in physical activity can effectively alleviate menopausal symptoms and enhance general well-being. Maintaining a healthy weight, bolstering bones, and elevating mood are all benefits.

Exercise Types to Incorporate:

Exercises for the heart: Cycling, swimming, and walking. Aim for 150 minutes or more a week of moderate to intense physical activity.

Strength training: Supports the preservation of bone density and muscle mass. Incorporate resistance band training or weightlifting twice a week.

Flexibility and Balance: Exercises like Pilates and yoga improve flexibility and lower the chance of falling.

Creating a routine

It might be difficult to include exercise and diet into a daily schedule, but doing so is essential for sustainability. Set reasonable initial goals and work your way up to greater duration and intensity.

Be consistent by creating a regular routine for your meals and exercise.

Variety: To keep things fresh and focus on various fitness-related topics, combine various exercise styles.

Support: To maintain your motivation, think about signing up for a fitness class or consulting a dietitian.

Stress Reduction with Mindfulness

Comprehending Mindfulness

Being mindful entails focusing on the here and now without passing judgment. It can lessen stress, lift one's spirits, and promote general wellbeing.

Applying Mindfulness:

Breathe mindfully by paying attention to your breath and inhaling and exhaling slowly and deeply.

Body Scan: Visualize a mental cross-section of your body, noting any tense spots.

Eating mindfully is taking in the flavor, texture, and aroma of your food while chewing carefully and appreciating every bite.

Techniques for Stress Management

The symptoms of menopause can be made worse by stress, so learning how to effectively handle it is crucial. Adding stress-reduction strategies to your regular routine can enhance your quality of life in general.

Meditation: Set aside a short period of time each day for guided meditation or introspection.

Physical Activity: Exercise can elevate mood and lower stress chemicals.

Social Networks: Keep up a robust support system of friends and relatives.

Combining Exercise and Mindfulness

Exercise and mindfulness can be improved by one another, with increased advantages for both physical and mental well-being.

Moving With Awareness:

Yoga: Blends breathing exercises with meditation and physical postures.

Tai Chi is a kind of mild martial arts that emphasizes deep breathing and calm, purposeful motions.

Walking meditation: Take a calm, deliberate stroll while paying attention to your legs and feet's sensations.

Goal-Setting for Long-Term Health

The Value of Establishing Goals

Establishing long-term health objectives gives one focus and inspiration. It assists you in tracking your development over time and maintaining focus on your general well-being.

Kinds of Health Objectives:

Short-Term Goals: Those that can be completed in a few weeks or months, such starting a new fitness regimen or dropping a certain amount of weight.

Long-Term Objectives: These might range from several months to years and include things like keeping a healthy weight, strengthening your heart, or eating a balanced diet.

SMART Goals Framework

Setting SMART goals can assist in defining specific, attainable objectives. SMART stands for Time-bound, Specific, Measurable, Achievable, and Relevant.

Setting SMART Objectives:

Particular: Clearly state your objective. Say "include five servings of fruits and vegetables daily" rather than "eat healthier."

Measurable: Make sure you can monitor your objective. As an illustration, "walk 10,000 steps a day."

Achievable: Make reasonable goals that complement your existing fitness level and way of living.

Relevant: Make decisions based on what's best for your general health.

Time-bound: Establish a due date for finishing your task.

Monitoring Development

You can maintain your motivation and make the required changes to your strategy by keeping a regular record of your progress.

Methods for Tracking Growth:

Journaling: Record your food, workouts, and mindfulness exercises in a health diary.

Apps: Track your dietary intake and exercise level with the help of fitness and health apps.

Frequent Check-ins: Plan on reviewing your goals on a regular basis and making any necessary adjustments.

Obstacles are unavoidable, but being prepared with tactics can help you stay on course.

Typical Problems and Their Fixes:

Lack of Time: Make time each day for exercise and meal preparation. Put your health first by seeing these appointments as non-negotiable.

Demotivation: To hold yourself accountable, find a workout partner or join a group. Establish modest incentives for hitting benchmarks.

Standstill: To keep things interesting, change up your routine. Try experimenting with new foods, workout routines, or mindfulness techniques.

Lisa's Path to Long-Term Wellness

During menopause, Lisa, a 49-year-old project manager, battled stress and weight gain. She developed a sustained healthy living plan by emphasizing exercise, mindfulness, and diet. Lisa began by establishing manageable objectives, such as increasing the amount of vegetables in her meals and going for daily walks. In order to cope with her stress, she also started doing yoga and mindfulness meditation.

Her physical and emotional well-being significantly improved as a result of these modest adjustments over time. Lisa's story demonstrates the value of handling menopause holistically.

Lisa's Success Tips

Start Small: To prevent feeling overwhelmed, concentrate on making one adjustment at a time.

Remain Adaptable: Show a readiness to modify your objectives and tactics as necessary.

Seek Support: Be in the company of encouraging friends and family.

During menopause, developing a sustained healthy living plan requires an all-encompassing strategy that includes goal-setting, regular exercise, mindfulness, and a balanced diet. You can enhance your overall quality of life and better manage menopausal symptoms by including these components into your everyday routine. Don't forget to monitor your progress, set reasonable targets, and adopt a flexible mindset. You may confidently handle menopause and embrace a healthier, more meaningful lifestyle with dedication and assistance.

Finally

Although there are particular difficulties associated with early menopause, it may also be a time of empowerment and good transformation if handled well. In order to successfully navigate this phase, "MenoPlay: Handling Early Menopause Hormonal Changes with Nutrition" equips you with the necessary knowledge and useful tools. This book provides thorough advice to help you manage your weight, temperament, sleep, and general health, from comprehending hormonal changes to putting good eating plans into practice.

Making wise decisions is essential to surviving the early menopause. You can enhance your quality of life and assist your body through hormonal changes by incorporating the dietary plans and lifestyle advice in this book. With confidence, accept the trip, knowing that you have what it takes to overcome the obstacles on the way to a happier, healthier future. Recall that menopause is a new chapter in your life rather than its end, and you can make the most of it if you have the necessary resources.